.

KETO VEGETARIAN COOKBOOK:

BREAKFAST RECIPES

Quick, Easy and Delicious Low Carb Recipes
for healthy living while keeping
your weight under control

Lisa Jackson

Copyright © 2021 by Lisa Jackson

TABLE OF CONTENTS

BREAKFAST RECIPES

Coffee Smoothie

Prep Time:5 minutes

Cook Time:0 minutes

Servings: 4

Ingredients:

- ➤ 4 cups baby spinach
- ➤ 4 tablespoons hemp hearts
- ➤ 12 Medjool dates, pitted
- ➤ 4 tablespoons cashew butter
- ➤ 2 cup brewed coffee, chilled
- ➤ 6 cups of ice cubes

Directions:

1. Place pitted dates in a medium bowl, cover with hot water and let them soak for 15 minutes.
2. Drain the dates, add them into a food processor along with the remaining ingredients, and then pulse for 1 to 2 minutes until blended, scraping the sides of the container frequently.

3. Distribute the smoothie among glasses and then serve.

   Nutrition: 391 Cal 15 g Fat 2 g Saturated Fat 60 g Carbohydrates 6 g Fiber 47 g Sugars 10 g Protein;

Banana Cream Pie and Chia Pudding

Prep Time:1 hour and 10 minutes

Cook Time:0 minutes

Servings: 4

Ingredients:

- ➤ 2 bananas, peeled, mashed
- ➤ 2 bananas, peeled, chopped
- ➤ 1/2 cup chia seeds
- ➤ 2 teaspoons cinnamon
- ➤ 4 tablespoons coconut flakes
- ➤ 1 cup coconut milk, unsweetened
- ➤ 2 tablespoons maple syrup
- ➤ 1 cup almond milk, unsweetened

Directions:

1. Take a large bowl, add chia seeds and mashed bananas, add maple syrup and cinnamon, pour in almond and coconut milk and then whisk until well combined.
2. Cover the bowl with lid, and then place it in the refrigerator for a minimum of 1 hour until firm.
3. When ready to eat, distribute pudding evenly among 4 bowls, top with chopped banana, and sprinkle with coconut flakes and then serve.

Nutrition: 350 Cal 17 g Fat 4 g Saturated Fat 37 g Carbohydrates 12 g Fiber 19 g Sugars 5 g Protein;

Brown Rice Breakfast Pudding

Prep Time:5 minutes

Cook Time:15 minutes

Servings: 4

Ingredients:

➢ 1 tart apple, cored, chopped

➢ 1 cup Medjool dates, pitted, chopped

➢ 3 cups cooked brown rice

➢ 1/8 teaspoon salt

➢ ¼ teaspoon ground cloves

➢ 1 cinnamon stick

➢ ¼ cup raisins

➢ ¼ cup slivered almonds, toasted

➢ 2 cups almond milk, unsweetened

Directions:

1. Take a medium saucepan, place it over medium-low heat, add rice, dates, cloves, and cinnamon, pour in milk, stir until mixed and cook for 12 minutes until thickened.

2. Then remove and discard cinnamon stick, add apple and raisins and then stir in salt.

3. Remove pan from heat, distribute pudding among four bowls and top with almonds.

4. Serve straight away.

Nutrition: 391 Cal 4.8 g Fat 0.6 g Saturated Fat 81.1 g Carbohydrates 5.7 g Fiber 24.8 g Sugars 6 g Protein;

Carrot Cake Oats

Prep Time:6 hours and 10 minutes

Cook Time:0 minutes

Servings: 4

Ingredients:

- ¼ cup shredded carrot
- 1/3 cup rolled oats
- 2 tablespoons chopped pineapple
- 1 tablespoon shredded coconut, unsweetened and more for topping
- 1 tablespoon ground flaxseed
- 1 tablespoon raisins and more for topping
- 2 tablespoons maple syrup and more for topping
- 1/8 teaspoon ground nutmeg
- ¼ teaspoon ground cinnamon and more for topping
- ¼ teaspoon vanilla extract, unsweetened
- 1 tablespoon chopped walnuts and more for topping
- ½ cup almond milk, unsweetened

Directions:

1. Take a large bowl, place all the ingredients in it, and stir until well mixed.

2. Cover the bowl with lid, and then place it in the refrigerator for a minimum of a minimum of 6 hours.

3. When ready to eat, distribute oats mixture evenly among 4 bowls, top with some shredded coconut, raisins, and walnuts, sprinkle with cinnamon, drizzle with maple syrup and then serve.

   Nutrition: 242 Cal 9 g Fat 2 g Saturated Fat 35 g Carbohydrates 6 g Fiber 12 g Sugars 7 g Protein;

Chocolate Chip and Coconut Pancakes

Prep Time:10 minutes

Cook Time:40 minutes

Servings: 8

Ingredients:

- 1¼ cups buckwheat flour
- 1 tablespoon flaxseeds
- 2 tablespoons coconut flakes, unsweetened
- ¼ cup rolled oats
- 1/8 teaspoon sea salt
- 1 tablespoon baking powder
- 1/3 cup mini chocolate chips, vegan
- ¼ cup maple syrup
- 1 teaspoon vanilla extract, unsweetened
- ½ cup applesauce, unsweetened
- 1 cup almond milk, unsweetened
- ½ cup of water
- 2 bananas, peeled, sliced

Directions:

1. Take a small saucepan, place it over medium heat, add flaxseeds, pour in water, and then cook for 4 to 5 minutes until sticky mixture comes together.

2. Strain the flaxseeds mixture immediately into a cup, discard the seeds, and set aside the collected flax water until required.

3. Take a large bowl, add buckwheat flour and oats in it, and then stir in salt, baking powder, and coconut until mixed.

4. Take a medium bowl, add 2 tablespoons of reserved flax water along with maple syrup and vanilla, pour in applesauce and milk, and whisk until combined.

5. Pour the milk mixture into the flour mixture, whisk well until thick batter comes together, and then fold in chocolate chips.

6. Take a griddle pan, place it over medium-low heat, spray it with oil and when hot, pour in 1/3 cup of the prepared batter, spread it gently and cook for 5 to 7 minutes until the bottom turns golden brown; pour in more batter if there is a space on the pan.

7. Flip the pancake, continue cooking for 5 minutes, and when done, transfer pancake to a plate and then repeat with the remaining batter.

8. Serve pancakes with sliced bananas.

Nutrition: 190 Cal 14 g Fat 6 g Saturated Fat 8 g Carbohydrates 2 g Fiber 4 g Sugars 8 g Protein;

Berries and Banana Smoothie Bowl

Prep Time:5 minutes

Cook Time:0 minutes

Servings: 4

Ingredients:

For the Smoothie:

➢ 4 cups frozen mixed berries

➢ 4 small frozen banana, sliced

➢ 4 scoops of vanilla protein powder

➢ 12 tablespoons almond milk, unsweetened

For the Toppings:

➢ 4 tablespoons chia seeds

➢ 4 tablespoons shredded coconut, unsweetened

➢ 4 tablespoons hemp seeds

➢ ½ cup Granola

➢ Fresh strawberries, sliced, as needed

Directions:

1. Add mixed berries into a food processor along with banana and then pulse at low speed for 1 to 2 minutes until broken.

2. Add remaining ingredients for the smoothie and then pulse again for 1 minute at low speed until

creamy, scraping the sides of the container frequently.

3. Distribute the smoothie among four bowls, then top with chia seeds, coconut, hemp seeds, granola, and strawberries and serve.

Nutrition: 214 Cal 2.5 g Fat 1.6 g Saturated Fat 47.5 g Carbohydrates 8.8 g Fiber 26 g Sugars 2.8 g Protein;

Mint Chocolate Protein Smoothie

Prep Time:5 minutes

Cook Time:0 minutes

Servings: 4

Ingredients:

- ➤ 4 tablespoons ground flaxseed
- ➤ 4 cups fresh spinach
- ➤ 4 frozen banana, sliced
- ➤ 4 scoops of chocolate protein powder
- ➤ 4 tablespoons chopped dark chocolate, vegan
- ➤ ½ cup melted dark chocolate
- ➤ 1 teaspoon peppermint extract, unsweetened
- ➤ 4 tablespoons honey
- ➤ 3 cups almond milk, unsweetened
- ➤ 1 cup ice cubed

Directions:

1. Add all the ingredients in the order into a food processor or blender and then pulse for 1 to 2 minutes until blended, scraping the sides of the container frequently.

2. Distribute the smoothie among glasses and then serve.

Nutrition: 480.5 Cal 20.3 g Fat 8.4 g Saturated Fat 45.6 g Carbohydrates 9.7 g Fiber 22.5 g Sugars 31.2 g Protein;

Sunrise Smoothie

Prep Time:5 minutes

Cook Time:0 minutes

Servings: 4

Ingredients:

- ➤ 4 tablespoons chia seed
- ➤ 2 frozen banana
- ➤ 2 lemon, peeled
- ➤ 2 cups diced carrots
- ➤ 4 clementine, peeled
- ➤ 4 cups frozen strawberries, unsweetened
- ➤ 12 tablespoons pomegranate tendrils
- ➤ 2 cup almond milk, unsweetened

Directions:

1. Add all the ingredients in the order into a food processor or blender and then pulse for 1 to 2 minutes until blended, scraping the sides of the container frequently.
2. Distribute the smoothie among glasses and then serve.

Nutrition: 274 Cal 5.4 g Fat 0.5 g Saturated Fat 57.3 g Carbohydrates 13.3 g Fiber 33.8 g Sugars 0.5 g Protein;

Sunshine Orange Smoothie

Prep Time:5 minutes

Cook Time:0 minutes

Servings: 4

Ingredients:

- ➤ 2 medium oranges, zested, juiced
- ➤ 4 frozen bananas
- ➤ 4 tablespoons goji berries
- ➤ ½ cup hemp seeds
- ➤ 1 teaspoon grated ginger
- ➤ 1 cup almond milk, unsweetened
- ➤ ½ cup of ice cubes

Directions:

1. Add all the ingredients in the order into a food processor or blender and then pulse for 1 to 2 minutes until blended, scraping the sides of the container frequently.
2. Distribute the smoothie among glasses and then serve.

Nutrition: 131 Cal 2.3 g Fat 0.3 g Saturated Fat 26.7 g Carbohydrates 4.4 g Fiber 11 g Sugars 2.6 g Protein;

Chocolate and Hazelnut Smoothie

Prep Time:5 minutes

Cook Time:0 minutes

Servings: 4

Ingredients:

- ➢ 1 frozen banana
- ➢ 1 cup hazelnuts, unsalted, roasted
- ➢ 8 teaspoons maple syrup
- ➢ 4 tablespoons cocoa powder, unsweetened
- ➢ 1/2 teaspoon hazelnut extract, unsweetened
- ➢ 2 cups almond milk, unsweetened
- ➢ 1 cup of ice cubes

Directions:

1. Add all the ingredients in the order into a food processor or blender and then pulse for 1 to 2 minutes until blended, scraping the sides of the container frequently.

2. Distribute the smoothie among glasses and then serve.

   Nutrition: 198 Cal 12 g Fat 1 g Saturated Fat 21 g Carbohydrates 5 g Fiber 12 g Sugars 5 g Protein;

Rainbow Taco Boats

Prep Time:10 minutes

Cook Time:0 minutes

Servings: 4 **Ingredients:**

- ➢ 1 head romaine lettuce, destemmed

  For the Filling:

- ➢ 1/2 cup alfalfa sprouts
- ➢ 1 medium avocado, peeled, pitted, cubed
- ➢ 1 cup shredded carrots
- ➢ 1 cup halved cherry tomatoes
- ➢ 3/4 cup sliced red cabbage
- ➢ 1/2 cup sprouted hummus dip
- ➢ 1 tablespoon hemp seeds

  For the Sauce:

- ➢ 1 tablespoon maple syrup
- ➢ 1/3 cup tahini
- ➢ 1/8 teaspoon sea salt
- ➢ 2 tablespoons lemon juice
- ➢ 3 tablespoons water

Directions:

1. Prepare the sauce and for this, take a medium bowl, add all the ingredients in it and whisk until well combined.

2. Assemble the boats and for this, arrange lettuce leaves in twelve portions, top each with hummus, and the remaining ingredients for the filling.

3. Serve with prepared sauce.

Nutrition: 314 Cal 23.6 g Fat 4 g Saturated Fat 23.2 g Carbohydrates 9.3 g Fiber 6.2 g Sugars 8 g Protein;

Eggplant Sandwich

Prep Time:10 minutes

Cook Time:25 minutes

Servings: 4

Ingredients:

For the Sandwich:

> 2 ciabatta buns
> 1 medium eggplant, peeled, sliced, soaked in salted water
> 1 medium tomato, sliced
> 1/2 of a medium cucumber, sliced
> 1/2 cup arugula
> 4 tablespoons mayo

For the Marinade:

> 1 teaspoon agave syrup
> 1/4 teaspoon salt
> 1/4 teaspoon ground black pepper
> 1 teaspoon smoked paprika
> 1 tablespoon soy sauce
> 1 tablespoon olive oil

Directions:

1. Switch on the oven, then set it to 350 degrees F and let it preheat.

2. Prepare the marinade and for this, take a small bowl, place all the ingredients in it and whisk until combined.

3. Drain the eggplant slices, pat dry with a kitchen towel, and brush with prepared marinade, arrange them on a baking sheet and then bake for 20 minutes until done.

4. Assemble the sandwich and for this, slice the bread in half lengthwise, then spread mayonnaise in the bottom half of the bun and top with baked eggplant slices, tomato, and cucumber slices, and sprinkle with salt and black pepper.

5. Top with arugula leaves, cover with the top half of the bun, and then cover with aluminum foil.

6. Preheat the grill over medium-high heat setting and when hot, place prepared sandwiches and grill for 3 to 5 minutes until toasted.

7. Cut each sandwich through the foil into half and serve.

Nutrition: 688 Cal 15 g Fat 2 g Saturated Fat 118 g Carbohydrates 7 g Fiber 7 g Sugars 21 g Protein;

Lentil, Cauliflower and Grape Salad

Prep Time:10 minutes

Cook Time:25 minutes

Servings: 4

Ingredients:

> For the Cauliflower:
> 1 medium head of cauliflower, cut into florets
> 1/4 teaspoon sea salt
> 1 1/2 tablespoons curry powder
> 1 1/2 tablespoons melted coconut oil

For the Tahini Dressing:

> 2 tablespoons tahini
> 1/8 teaspoon salt
> 1.8 teaspoon ground black pepper
> 4 1/2 tablespoons green curry paste
> 1 tablespoon maple syrup
> 2 tablespoons lemon juice
> 2 tablespoons water

For the Salad:

> 1 cup cooked lentils
> 4 tablespoons chopped cilantro
> 1 cup red grapes, halved
> 6 cups mixed greens

Directions:

1. Switch on the oven, then set it to 400 degrees F and let it preheat.
2. Prepare the cauliflower and for this, take a medium bowl, place cauliflower florets in it, drizzle with oil, season with salt and curry powder, toss until mixed.
3. Take a baking sheet, line it with parchment sheet, spread cauliflower florets in it, and then bake for 25 minutes until tender and nicely golden brown.
4. Meanwhile, prepare the tahini dressing and for this, take a medium bowl, place all of its ingredients and whisk until combined, set aside until required.
5. Assemble the salad and for this, take a large salad bowl, add roasted cauliflower florets, lentils, grapes, and mixed greens, drizzle with prepared tahini dressing and toss until well combined.
6. Serve straight away.

Nutrition: 420 Cal 14 g Fat 5 g Saturated Fat 37.6 g Carbohydrates 9.8 g Fiber 12.8 g Sugars 10.8 g Protein;

Loaded Kale Salad

Prep Time: **10 minutes**

Cook Time: 30 minutes

Servings: 4

Ingredients:

- 1 ½ cup cooked quinoa
  For The Vegetables:
- 1 whole beet, peeled, sliced
- 4 large carrots, peeled, chopped
- 1/2 teaspoon curry powder
- 1/8 teaspoon sea salt
- 2 tablespoons melted coconut oil
  For The Dressing:
- ¼ teaspoon of sea salt
- 2 tablespoons maple syrup
- 3 tablespoons lemon juice
- 1/3 cup tahini
- 1/4 cup water
  For the Salad:
- 1/2 cup sprouts
- 1 medium avocado, peeled, pitted, cubed
- 1/2 cup chopped cherry tomatoes
- 8 cups chopped kale

➢ 1/4 cup hemp seeds

Directions:

1. Switch on the oven, then set it to 375 degrees F and let it preheat.

2. Take a baking sheet, place beets and carrots on it, drizzle with oil, season with curry powder and salt, toss until coated, and then bake for 30 minutes until tender and golden brown.

3. Meanwhile, prepare the dressing and for this, take a small bowl, place all the ingredients in it and whisk until well combined, set aside until required.

4. Assemble the salad and for this, take a large salad bowl, place kale leaves in it, add remaining ingredients for the salad along with roasted vegetables, drizzle with prepared dressing and toss until combined.

5. Serve straight away.

Nutrition: 472 Cal 22.8 g Fat 3.8 g Saturated Fat 58.7 g Carbohydrates 12.5 g Fiber 9.2 g Sugars 14.6 g Protein;

Tuna Salad

Prep Time:10 minutes

Cook Time:0 minutes

Servings: 4

Ingredients:

➢ 1/2 cup chopped celery

➢ 3 cups cooked chickpeas

➢ 1 tablespoon capers, chopped

➢ 2 tablespoons sweet pickle relish

➢ 1 tablespoon yellow mustard paste

➢ 2 tablespoons mayonnaise

Directions:

1. Take a medium bowl, place chickpeas in it, add mustard and mayonnaise and mash by using a fork until peas are broken.

2. Add remaining ingredients and stir until well combined.

3. Serve straight away.

Nutrition: 207 Cal 7 g Fat 1 g Saturated Fat 27 g Carbohydrates 8 g Fiber 1 g Sugars 9 g Protein;

White Bean and Artichoke Sandwich

Prep Time:15 minutes

Cook Time:10 minutes

Servings: 4

Ingredients:

- ➢ 1 ¼ cooked white beans
- ➢ ½ cup cashew nuts
- ➢ 6 artichoke hearts, chopped
- ➢ ¼ cup sunflower seeds, hulled
- ➢ 1 clove of garlic, peeled
- ➢ ¼ teaspoon salt
- ➢ ¼ teaspoon ground black pepper
- ➢ 1 teaspoon dried rosemary
- ➢ 1 lemon, grated
- ➢ 6 tablespoons almond milk, unsweetened
- ➢ 8 pieces of rustic bread

Directions:

1. Soak cashew nuts in warm water for 10 minutes, then drain them and transfer into a food processor.

2. Add garlic, salt, black pepper, rosemary, lemon zest, and milk and then pulse for 2 minutes until

smooth, scraping the sides of the container frequently.

3. Take a medium bowl, place beans in it, mash them by using a fork, then add sunflower seeds and artichokes and stir until mixed.

4. Pour in cashew nuts dressing, stir until coated, and taste to adjust seasoning.

5. Take a medium skillet pan, place it over medium heat, add bread slices, and cook for 3 minutes per side until toasted.

6. Spread white beans mixture on one side of four bread slices and then cover with the other four slices.

7. Serve straight away.

Nutrition: 220 Cal 8 g Fat 1 g Saturated Fat 28 g Carbohydrates 8 g Fiber 2 g Sugars 12 g Protein;

Sabich Sandwich

Prep Time:10 minutes

Cook Time:10 minutes

Servings: 4

Ingredients:

- ➢ 1/2 cup cooked white beans
- ➢ 2 medium potatoes, peeled, boiled, ½-inch thick sliced
- ➢ 1 medium eggplant, destemmed, ½-inch cubed
- ➢ 4 dill pickles, ¼-inch thick sliced
- ➢ ¼ teaspoon of sea salt
- ➢ 2 tablespoons olive oil
- ➢ 1/4 teaspoon harissa paste
- ➢ 1/2 cup hummus
- ➢ 1 tablespoon mayonnaise
- ➢ 4 pita bread pockets
- ➢ 1/2 cup tabbouleh salad

Directions:

1. Take a small frying pan, place it over medium-low heat, add oil and wait until it gets hot.
2. Season eggplant pieces with salt, add to the hot frying pan and cook for 8 minutes until softened, and when done, remove the pan from heat.

3. Take a small bowl, place white beans in it, add harissa paste and mayonnaise and then stir until combined.

4. Assemble the sandwich and for this, place pita bread on clean working space, smear generously with hummus, then cover half of each pita bread with potato slices and top with a dill pickle slices.

5. Spoon 2 tablespoons of white bean mixture on each dill pickle, top with 3 tablespoons of cooked eggplant pieces and 2 tablespoons of tabbouleh salad and then cover the filling with the other half of pita bread.

6. Serve straight away.

Nutrition: 386 Cal 13 g Fat 2 g Saturated Fat 56 g Carbohydrates 7 g Fiber 3 g Sugars 12 g Protein;

Chickpea and Mayonnaise Salad Sandwich

Prep Time:10 minutes

Cook Time:0 minutes

Servings: 4

Ingredients:

For the mayonnaise:

- 1/3 cup cashew nuts, soaked in boiling water for 10 minutes
- ½ teaspoon ground black pepper
- 1 teaspoon salt
- 6 teaspoons apple cider vinegar
- 2 teaspoon maple syrup
- 1/2 teaspoon Dijon mustard

For the chickpea salad:

- 1 small bunch of chives, chopped
- 1 ½ cup sweetcorn
- 3 cups cooked chickpeas
  To serve:
- 4 sandwich bread
- 4 leaves of lettuce
- ½ cup chopped cherry tomatoes

Directions:

1. Prepare the mayonnaise and for this, place all of its ingredients in a food processor and then pulse for 2 minutes until smooth, scraping the sides of the container frequently.
2. Take a medium bowl, place chickpeas in it, and then mash by using a fork until broken.
3. Add chives and corn, stir until mixed, then add mayonnaise and stir until well combined.
4. Assemble the sandwich and for this, stuff sandwich bread with chickpea salad, top each sandwich with a lettuce leaf, and ¼ cup of chopped tomatoes and then serve.

Nutrition: 387 Cal 19 g Fat 5 g Saturated Fat 39.7 g Carbohydrates 7.2 g Fiber 4.6 g Sugars 10 g Protein;

Grilled Avocado Guacamole

Prep Time:10 minutes

Cook Time:20 minutes

Servings: 4

Ingredients:

- ½ teaspoon olive oil
- 1 lime, halved
- ½ onion, halved
- 1 serrano chile, halved, stemmed, and seeded
- 3 Haas avocados, skin on
- 2–3 tablespoons fresh cilantro, chopped
- ½ teaspoon smoked salt

Directions:

1. Preheat the grill over medium heat.
2. Brush the grilling grates with olive oil and place chile, onion, and lime on it.
3. Grill the onion for 10 minutes, chile for 5 minutes, and lime for 2 minutes.
4. Transfer the veggies to a large bowl.
5. Now cut the avocados in half and grill them for 5 minutes.
6. Mash the flesh of the grilled avocado in a bowl.

7. Chop the other grilled veggies and add them to the avocado mash.
8. Stir in remaining ingredients and mix well.
9. Serve.

Nutrition: Calories: 165 Total Fat: 17g Carbs: 4g Net Carbs: 2g Fiber: 1g Protein: 1g

Tofu Hoagie Rolls

Prep Time: 10 minutes

Cook Time:20 minutes

Servings: 6

Ingredients:

- ➤ ½ cup vegetable broth
- ➤ ¼ cup hot sauce
- ➤ 1 tablespoon vegan butter
- ➤ 1 (16 ounce) package tofu, pressed and diced
- ➤ 4 cups cabbage, shredded
- ➤ 2 medium apples, grated
- ➤ 1 medium shallot, grated
- ➤ 6 tablespoons vegan mayonnaise
- ➤ 1 tablespoon apple cider vinegar
- ➤ Salt and black pepper
- ➤ 4 6-inch hoagie rolls, toasted

Directions:

1. In a saucepan, combine broth with butter and hot sauce and bring to a boil.
2. Add tofu and reduce the heat to a simmer.
3. Cook for 10 minutes then remove from heat and let sit for 10 minutes to marinate.

4. Toss cabbage and rest of the ingredients in a salad bowl.

5. Prepare and set up a grill on medium heat.

6. Drain the tofu and grill for 5 minutes per side.

7. Lay out the toasted hoagie rolls and add grilled tofu to each hoagie

8. Add the cabbage mixture evenly between them then close it.

9. Serve.

Nutrition: Calories: 111 Total Fat: 11g Carbs: 5g Net Carbs: 1g Fiber: 0g Protein: 1g

Grilled Seitan with Creole Sauce

Prep Time: 10 minutes

Cook Time:14 minutes

Servings: 4

Ingredients:

Grilled Seitan Kebabs:

- 4 cups seitan, diced
- 2 medium onions, diced into squares
- 8 bamboo skewers
- 1 can coconut milk
- 2½ tablespoons creole spice
- 2 tablespoons tomato paste
- 2 cloves of garlic

  Creole Spice Mix:

- 2 tablespoons paprika
- 12 dried peri chili peppers
- 1 tablespoon salt
- 1 tablespoon freshly ground pepper
- 2 teaspoons dried thyme
- 2 teaspoons dried oregano

Directions:

1. Prepare the creole seasoning by blending all its ingredients and preserve in a sealable jar.

2. Thread seitan and onion on the bamboo skewers in an alternating pattern.
3. On a baking sheet, mix coconut milk with creole seasoning, tomato paste and garlic.
4. Soak the skewers in the milk marinade for 2 hours.
5. Prepare and set up a grill over medium heat.
6. Grill the skewers for 7 minutes per side.
7. Serve.

Nutrition: Calories: 407 Total Fat: 42g Carbs: 13g Net Carbs: 6g Fiber: 1g Protein: 4g

Mushroom Steaks

Prep Time: 10 minutes

Cook Time:24 minutes

Servings: 4

Ingredients:

- ➢ 1 tablespoon vegan butter
- ➢ ½ cup vegetable broth
- ➢ ½ small yellow onion, diced
- ➢ 1 large garlic clove, minced
- ➢ 3 tablespoons balsamic vinegar
- ➢ 1 tablespoon mirin
- ➢ ½ tablespoon soy sauce
- ➢ ½ tablespoon tomato paste
- ➢ 1 teaspoon dried thyme
- ➢ ½ teaspoon dried basil
- ➢ A dash of ground black pepper
- ➢ 2 large, whole portobello mushrooms

Directions:

1. Melt butter in a saucepan over medium heat and stir in half of the broth.

2. Bring to a simmer then add garlic and onion. Cook for 8 minutes.

3. Whisk the rest of the ingredients except the mushrooms in a bowl.

4. Add this mixture to the onion in the pan and mix well.

5. Bring this filling to a simmer then remove from the heat.

6. Clean the mushroom caps inside and out and divide the filling between the mushrooms.

7. Place the mushrooms on a baking sheet and top them with remaining sauce and broth.

8. Cover with foil then place it on a grill to smoke.

9. Cover the grill and broil for 16 minutes over indirect heat. Serve warm.

Nutrition: Calories: 887 Total Fat: 93g Carbs: 29g Net Carbs: 13g Fiber: 4g Protein: 8g

Grilled Portobello

Prep Time: 10 minutes

Cook Time:8 minutes

Servings: 4

Ingredients:

- ➢ 4 portobello mushrooms
- ➢ ¼ cup soy sauce
- ➢ ¼ cup tomato sauce
- ➢ 2 tablespoons maple syrup
- ➢ 1 tablespoon molasses
- ➢ 2 tablespoons minced garlic
- ➢ 1 tablespoon onion powder
- ➢ 1 pinch salt and pepper

Directions:

1. Mix all the ingredients except mushrooms in a bowl.
2. Add mushrooms to this marinade and mix well to coat.
3. Cover and marinate for 1 hour.
4. Prepare and set up the grill at medium heat. Grease it with cooking spray.
5. Grill the mushroom for 4 minutes per side.
6. Serve

Nutrition: Calories: 404 Total Fat: 43g Carbs: 8g Net Carbs: 4g Fiber: 1g Protein: 4g

Wok Fried Broccoli

Prep Time: 10 minutes

Cook Time:16 minutes

Servings: 2

Ingredients:

- ➤ 3 ounces whole, blanched peanuts
- ➤ 2 tablespoons olive oil
- ➤ 1 banana shallot, sliced
- ➤ 10 ounces broccoli, trimmed and cut into florets
- ➤ ¼ red pepper, julienned
- ➤ ½ yellow pepper, julienned
- ➤ 1 teaspoon soy sauce

Directions:

1. Toast peanuts on a baking sheet for 15 minutes at 350 degrees F.
2. In a wok, add oil and shallots and sauté for 10 minutes.
3. Toss in broccoli and peppers.
4. Stir fry for 3 minutes then add the rest of the ingredients.
5. Cook for 3 additional minutes and serve.

Nutrition: Calories: 391 Total Fat: 39g Carbs: 15g Net Carbs: 5g Fiber: 2g Protein: 6g

Broccoli & Brown Rice Satay

Prep Time: 10 minutes

Cook Time:10 minutes

Servings: 4

Ingredients:

- ➢ 6 trimmed broccoli florets, halved
- ➢ 1-inch piece of ginger, shredded
- ➢ 2 garlic cloves, shredded
- ➢ 1 red onion, sliced
- ➢ 1 roasted red pepper, cut into cubes
- ➢ 2 teaspoons olive oil
- ➢ 1 teaspoon mild chili powder
- ➢ 1 tablespoon reduced salt soy sauce
- ➢ 1 tablespoon maple syrup
- ➢ 1 cup cooked brown rice

Directions:

1. Boil broccoli in water for 4 minutes then drain immediately.
2. In a pan add olive oil, ginger, onion, and garlic.
3. Stir fry for 2 minutes then add the rest of the ingredients.
4. Cook for 3 minutes then serve.

Nutrition: Calories: 196 Total Fat: 20g Carbs: 8g
Net Carbs: 3g Fiber: 1g Protein: 3g

Sautéed Sesame Spinach

Prep Time: 1 hr. 10 minutes

Cook Time:3 minutes

Servings: 4

Ingredients:

- ➢ 1 tablespoon toasted sesame oil
- ➢ ½ tablespoon soy sauce
- ➢ ½ teaspoon toasted sesame seeds, crushed
- ➢ ½ teaspoon rice vinegar
- ➢ ½ teaspoon golden caster sugar
- ➢ 1 garlic clove, grated
- ➢ 8 ounces spinach, stem ends trimmed

Directions:

1. Sauté spinach in a pan until it is wilted.
2. Whisk the sesame oil, garlic, sugar, vinegar, sesame seeds, soy sauce and black pepper together in a bowl.
3. Stir in spinach and mix well.
4. Cover and refrigerate for 1 hour.
5. Serve.

   Nutrition: Calories: 677 Total Fat: 60g Carbs: 71g Net Carbs: 7g Fiber: 0g; Protein: 20g

SMOOTHIES AND BEVERAGES

Kale Smoothie

Prep Time:5 minutes

Cook Time:0 minutes

Servings: 2

Ingredients:

> 2 cups chopped kale leaves
> 1 banana, peeled
> 1 cup frozen strawberries
> 1 cup unsweetened almond milk
> 4 Medjool dates, pitted and chopped

Directions:

1. Put all the ingredients in a food processor, then blitz until glossy and smooth.
2. Serve immediately or chill in the refrigerator for an hour before serving.

Nutrition: Calories: 663 Fat: 10.0g Carbs: 142.5g Fiber: 19.0g Protein: 17.4g

Hot Tropical Smoothie

Prep Time:5 minutes

Cook Time:0 minutes

Servings: **4**

Ingredients:

- ➢ 1 cup frozen mango chunks
- ➢ 1 cup frozen pineapple chunks
- ➢ 1 small tangerine, peeled and pitted
- ➢ 2 cups spinach leaves
- ➢ 1 cup coconut water
- ➢ ¼ teaspoon cayenne pepper, optional

Directions:

1. Add all the ingredients in a food processor, then blitz until the mixture is smooth and combine well.
2. Serve immediately or chill in the refrigerator for an hour before serving.

Nutrition: Calories: 283 Fat: 1.9g Carbs: 67.9g Fiber: 10.4g Protein: 6.4g

Cranberry and Banana Smoothie

Prep Time:5 minutes

Cook Time:0 minutes

Servings: 4

- ➢ 1 cup frozen cranberries
- ➢ 1 large banana, peeled
- ➢ 4 Medjool dates, pitted and chopped
- ➢ 1½ cups unsweetened almond milk

Directions:

1. Add all the ingredients in a food processor, then process until the mixture is glossy and well mixed.

2. Serve immediately or chill in the refrigerator for an hour before serving.

Nutrition: Calories: 616 Fat: 8.0g Carbs: 132.8g Fiber: 14.6g Protein: 15.7g

Super Smoothie

Prep Time:5 minutes

Cook Time:0 minutes

Servings: 4

Ingredients:

- ➢ 1 banana, peeled
- ➢ 1 cup chopped mango
- ➢ 1 cup raspberries
- ➢ ¼ cup rolled oats
- ➢ 1 carrot, peeled
- ➢ 1 cup chopped fresh kale
- ➢ 2 tablespoons chopped fresh parsley
- ➢ 1 tablespoon flaxseeds
- ➢ 1 tablespoon grated fresh ginger
- ➢ ½ cup unsweetened soy milk
- ➢ 1 cup water

Directions:

1. Put all the ingredients in a food processor, then blitz until glossy and smooth.
2. Serve immediately or chill in the refrigerator for an hour before serving.

Nutrition: Calories: 550 Fat: 39.0g Carbs: 31.0g Fiber: 15.0g Protein: 13.0g

Light Ginger Tea

Prep Time:5 minutes

Cook Time:10 to 15 minutes

Servings: 2

Ingredients:

➤ 1 small ginger knob, sliced into four 1-inch chunks

➤ 4 cups water

➤ Juice of 1 large lemon

➤ Maple syrup, to taste

Directions:

1. Add the ginger knob and water in a saucepan, then simmer over medium heat for 10 to 15 minutes.

2. Turn off the heat, then mix in the lemon juice. Strain the liquid to remove the ginger, then fold in the maple syrup and serve.

Nutrition: Calories: 32 Fat: 0.1g Carbs: 8.6g Fiber: 0.1g Protein: 0.1g

Lime and Cucumber Electrolyte Drink

Prep Time:5 minutes

Cook Time:0 minutes

Servings: **4**

Ingredients:

- ¼ cup chopped cucumber
- 1 tablespoon fresh lime juice
- 1 tablespoon apple cider vinegar
- 2 tablespoons maple syrup
- ¼ teaspoon sea salt, optional
- 4 cups water

Directions:

1. Combine all the ingredients in a glass. Stir to mix well.
2. Refrigerate overnight before serving.

Nutrition: Calories: 114 Fat: 0.1g Carbs: 28.9g Fiber: 0.3g Protein: 0.3g

Simple Date Shake

Prep Time:10 minutes

Cook Time:0 minutes

Servings: **2**

Ingredients:

> 5 Medjool dates, pitted, soaked in boiling water for 5 minutes
> ¾ cup unsweetened coconut milk
> 1 teaspoon vanilla extract
> ½ teaspoon fresh lemon juice
> ¼ teaspoon sea salt, optional
> 1½ cups ice

Directions:

1. Put all the ingredients in a food processor, then blitz until it has a milkshake and smooth texture.
2. Serve immediately.

Nutrition: Calories: 380 Fat: 21.6g Carbs: 50.3g Fiber: 6.0g Protein: 3.2g

Beet and Clementine Protein Smoothie

Prep Time:10 minutes

Cook Time:0 minutes

Servings: **3**

Ingredients:

➢ 1 small beet, peeled and chopped

➢ 1 clementine, peeled and broken into segments

➢ ½ ripe banana

➢ ½ cup raspberries

➢ 1 tablespoon chia seeds

➢ 2 tablespoons almond butter

➢ ¼ teaspoon vanilla extract

➢ 1 cup unsweetened almond milk

➢ 1/8 teaspoon fine sea salt, optional

Directions:

1. Combine all the ingredients in a food processor, then pulse on high for 2 minutes or until glossy and creamy.

2. Refrigerate for an hour and serve chilled.

Nutrition: Calories: 526 Fat: 25.4g Carbs: 61.9g Fiber: 17.3g Protein: 20.6g

Matcha Limeade

Prep Time:10 minutes

Cook Time:0 minutes

Servings: 4

Ingredients:

- ➢ 2 tablespoons matcha powder
- ➢ ¼ cup raw agave syrup
- ➢ 3 cups water, divided
- ➢ 1 cup fresh lime juice
- ➢ 3 tablespoons chia seeds

Directions:

1. Lightly simmer the matcha, agave syrup, and 1 cup of water in a saucepan over medium heat. Keep stirring until no matcha lumps.
2. Pour the matcha mixture in a large glass, then add the remaining ingredients and stir to mix well.
3. Refrigerate for at least an hour before serving.

Nutrition: Calories: 152 Fat: 4.5g Carbs: 26.8g Fiber: 5.3g Protein: 3.7g

Ambrosia with Pineapple

Prep Time:30 Minutes

Cook Time:15 Minutes

Servings: 4

Ingredients:

➤ Orange zest, two teaspoons

➤ Tofu, soft, pureed, one half cup

➤ Orange juice, three tablespoons

➤ Lemon juice, one third cup

➤ Cornstarch, one tablespoon

➤ Coconut, unsweetened shredded, one half cup

➤ Grapes, one cup

➤ Sugar, three tablespoons

➤ Strawberries, sliced, one cup

➤ Orange slices, one cup

➤ Apples, fresh sliced, one cup

➤ Pineapple, fresh chopped, one cup

Directions:

1. Use a large-sized bowl to assemble the fruits together and put it in the refrigerator.

2. In a small saucepan, mix together the lemon juice with the cornstarch and keep stirring until they are well mixed.

3. Add in the orange juice and the sugar and place the saucepan over medium-high heat. Cook the mix for five to ten minutes while the mixture gets thicker. Keep stirring constantly.

4. When the mixture is thick, then take the saucepan off of the heat and let it get completely cool.

5. When the mixture in the saucepan has cooled completely, then blends in the orange zest and the pureed tofu.

6. Allow this bowl of mix to rest in the refrigerator for one hour until it becomes chilled. Pour the dressing over the fruit before serving.

Nutrition: Calories: 257 Protein: 8g Fat: 8g Carbs: 44g

Tropical Fruit Salad

Prep Time:10 Minutes

Cook Time:0 Minutes

Servings: 2

Ingredients:

- Lime juice, one tablespoon
- Kiwi, two
- Dragon fruit, one half of one
- Strawberries, twelve
- Mango, one half of one

Directions:

1. Peel the fruits and chop them into bite-sized pieces. Dump all of the fruit chunks into a large-sized mixing bowl.
2. Drizzle the lime juice over the fruit and toss the fruit gently to coat all of the pieces with the juice. Serve immediately

Nutrition: Calories: 154 Protein: 2g Fat: 1g Carbs: 37g

Fall Fruit with Creamy Dressing

Prep Time:25 Minutes

Cook Time:0 Minutes

Servings: **4**

Ingredients:

Salad

> ➢ Pumpkin, raw, shredded, one half cup
> ➢ Pomegranate seeds, one half cup
> ➢ Grapes, one cup
> ➢ Apples, three, cored and cubed
>   Creamy Dressing
> ➢ Cinnamon, one teaspoon
> ➢ Lemon juice, one tablespoon
> ➢ Almond yogurt, one half cup

Directions:

1. Mix together all of the listed Ingredients for the dressing.
2. In a large-sized bowl, toss the dressing with the shredded raw pumpkin, pomegranate seeds, apples, and the dressing. Serve immediately.

   Nutrition: Calories: 161 Protein: 3g Fat: 1g Carbs: 40g

Fruit Salad with Sweet Lime Dressing

Prep Time:15 Minutes

Cook Time:0 Minutes

Servings: 9

Ingredients:

Salad

- Mint, fresh chopped, one cup
- Lime juice, two tablespoons
- Kiwi, five, peeled and sliced
- Mangoes, two, peeled and chopped
- Green grapes, one cup cut in half
- Blackberries, one cup
- Blueberries, one cup
- Strawberries, one cup sliced

  Sweet Lime Dressing

- Powdered sugar, two tablespoons
- Lime juice, two tablespoons

Directions:

1. Mix together until smooth in a small-sized bowl the powdered sugar and the lime juice.
2. Mix together in a large-sized bowl the fruits, then pour on the dressing and gently toss all of the fruits together well to coat all of the pieces.

3. This will stay good in the refrigerator for no more than one day.

Nutrition: Calories: 50 Protein: 1g Fat: 1g Carbs: 12g

Asian Fruit Salad

Prep Time:30 Minutes

Cook Time:0 Minutes

Servings: 8

Ingredients:

- Passion fruit, one-half cup (about six of the fruit)
- Papaya, one chopped
- Pineapple, one cup chunked
- Oranges, two separated into segments
- Star fruit, three sliced thin
- Mangoes, two large, peeled and chunked
- Mint, fresh, one-third cup chopped coarse
- Lime juice, one third cup
- Lime zest, one tablespoon
- Ginger, ground, one tablespoon
- Vanilla extract, one tablespoon
- Brown sugar, one half cup
- Water, four cups

Directions:

1. Mix the water and the sugar together in a medium-sized saucepan and put it over a medium to high heat until the sugar is dissolved.

2. Let this simmer for five minutes over a very low heat, so the sugar does not burn. Add in the vanilla extract and the ginger and stir well.

3. Let this cook for ten more minutes. Let the mix cool off the heat until it is room temperature, and then add in the mint, juice, and zest.

4. During the time the sauce is cooling mix together the remainder of the Ingredients in a large-sized bowl.

5. Pour the syrup mixture over the fruit in the bowl and mix gently to coat all pieces with the sauce.

6. Put the bowl in the refrigerator until the fruit is cold then serve.

Nutrition: Calories: 220 Protein: 3g Fat: 1g Carbs: 56g

Mimosa Salad

Prep Time:10 Minutes

Cook Time:0 Minutes

Servings: **8**

Ingredients:

- ➤ Mint, fresh, one half cup
- ➤ Orange juice, one half cup
- ➤ Pineapple, one cup cut into small pieces
- ➤ Strawberries, one cup cut into quarters
- ➤ Blueberries, one cup
- ➤ Blackberries, one cup
- ➤ Kiwi, three peeled and sliced

Directions:

1. In a large-sized bowl, mix all of the fruits together and then top with the orange juice and the fresh mint.
2. Toss gently together all of the fruit until they are well mixed.

Nutrition: Calories: 215 Protein: 3g Fat: 1g Carbs: 49g

Honey Lime Quinoa Fruit Salad

Prep Time:20 Minutes

Cook Time:0 Minutes

Servings: 6

Ingredients:

- Basil, chopped, one tablespoon
- Lime juice, two tablespoons
- Mango, diced, one cup
- Blueberries, one cup
- Blackberries, one cup
- Strawberries, sliced, one and one half cup
- Quinoa, cooked, one cup

Directions:

1. In a large-sized bowl, mix the fruits with the cooked quinoa and mix well.
2. Drizzle on the lime juice and add the chopped basil and mix the fruit gently but thoroughly to coat all of the pieces.

Nutrition: Calories: 246 Protein: 7g Fat: 1g Carbs: 44g

Chocolate Banana Shake

Prep Time:10 minutes

Cook Time:10 minutes

Servings: 2

Ingredients:

- ➢ 2 medium frozen bananas, peeled
- ➢ 4 dates, pitted
- ➢ 4 tablespoons peanut butter
- ➢ 4 tablespoons rolled oats
- ➢ 2 tablespoons cacao powder
- ➢ 2 tablespoons chia seeds
- ➢ 2 cups unsweetened soymilk

Directions:

1. Place all the ingredients in a high-speed blender and pulse until creamy.

2. Pour into two glasses and serve immediately.

Nutrition: Calories: 502 Fat: 4g Protein: 11g Sugar: 9g

Fruity Tofu Smoothie

Prep Time:10 minutes

Cook Time:10 minutes

Servings: 2

Ingredients:

- ➢ 12 ounces silken tofu, pressed and drained
- ➢ 2 medium bananas, peeled
- ➢ 1½ cups fresh blueberries
- ➢ 1 tablespoon maple syrup
- ➢ 1½ cups unsweetened soymilk
- ➢ ¼ cup ice cubes

Directions:

1. Place all the ingredients in a high-speed blender and pulse until creamy.
2. Pour into two glasses and serve immediately.

Nutrition: Calories 235 Carbohydrates: 1.9g Protein: 14.3g Fat: 18.9g

Protein Latte

Prep Time:10 minutes

Cook Time:10 minutes

Servings: 2

Ingredients:

- ➢ 2 cups hot brewed coffee
- ➢ 1¼ cups coconut milk
- ➢ 2 teaspoons coconut oil
- ➢ 2 scoops unsweetened vegan vanilla protein powder

Directions:

1. Place all the ingredients in a high-speed blender and pulse until creamy.
2. Pour into two serving mugs and serve immediately.

Nutrition: Calories 483 Carbs: 5.2g Protein: 45.2g Fat: 31.2g

Thai Iced Tea

Prep Time:5 minutes

Cook Time:10 minutes

Servings: 4

Ingredients:

- ➢ 4 cups of water
- ➢ 1 can of light coconut milk (14 oz.)
- ➢ ¼ cup of maple syrup
- ➢ ¼ cup of muscovado sugar
- ➢ 1 teaspoon of vanilla extract
- ➢ 2 tablespoons of loose-leaf black tea

Directions:

1. In a large saucepan, over medium heat bring the water to a boil.
2. Turn off the heat and add in the tea, cover and let steep for five minutes.
3. Strain the tea into a bowl or jug. Add the maple syrup, muscovado sugar, and vanilla extract. Give it a good whisk to blend all the ingredients together.
4. Set in the refrigerator to chill. Upon serving, pour ¾ of the tea into each glass, top with coconut milk and stir.

Tips:

Add a shot of dark rum to turn this iced tea into a cocktail.

You could substitute the coconut milk for almond or rice milk too.

Nutrition: Calories 844 Carbohydrates: 2.3g Protein: 21.6g Fat: 83.1g

Hibiscus Tea

Prep Time:1 Minute

Cook Time:5 minutes

Servings: 2 servings

Ingredients:

- ➢ 1 tablespoon of raisins, diced
- ➢ 6 Almonds, raw and unsalted
- ➢ ½ teaspoon of hibiscus powder
- ➢ 2 cups of water

Directions:

1. Bring the water to a boil in a small saucepan, add in the hibiscus powder and raisins. Give it a good stir, cover and let simmer for a further two minutes.

2. Strain into a teapot and serve with a side helping of almonds.

Tips:

As an alternative to this tea, do not strain it and serve with the raisin pieces still swirling around in the teacup.

You could also serve this tea chilled for those hotter days.

Double or triple the recipe to provide you with iced-tea to enjoy during the week without having to make a fresh pot each time.

Nutrition: Calories 139 Carbohydrates: 2.7g Protein: 8.7g Fat: 10.3

Lemon and Rosemary Iced Tea

Prep Time:5 minutes

Cook Time:10 minutes

Servings: 4 servings

Ingredients:

- ➢ 4 cups of water
- ➢ 4 earl grey tea bags
- ➢ ¼ cup of sugar
- ➢ 2 lemons
- ➢ 1 sprig of rosemary

Directions:

1. Peel the two lemons and set the fruit aside.
2. In a medium saucepan, over medium heat combine the water, sugar, and lemon peels. Bring this to a boil.
3. Remove from the heat and place the rosemary and tea into the mixture. Cover the saucepan and steep for five minutes.
4. Add the juice of the two peeled lemons to the mixture, strain, chill, and serve.

Tips: Skip the sugar and use honey to taste.

Do not squeeze the tea bags as they can cause the tea to become bitter.

Nutrition: Calories 229 Carbs: 33.2g Protein: 31.1g Fat: 10.2g

Lavender and Mint Iced Tea

Prep Time:5 minutes

Cook Time:10 minutes

Servings: 8 servings

Ingredients:

- 8 cups of water
- 1/3 cup of dried lavender buds
- ¼ cup of mint

Directions:

1. Add the mint and lavender to a pot and set this aside.
2. Add in eight cups of boiling water to the pot. Sweeten to taste, cover and let steep for ten minutes. Strain, chill, and serve.

Tips:

Use a sweetener of your choice when making this iced tea.

Add spirits to turn this iced tea into a summer cocktail.

Nutrition: Calories 266 Carbs: 9.3g Protein: 20.9g Fat: 16.1g

Energizing Ginger Detox Tonic

Prep Time:15 minutes

Cook Time:10 minutes

Servings:

Ingredients:

➢ 1/2 teaspoon of grated ginger, fresh

➢ 1 small lemon slice

➢ 1/8 teaspoon of cayenne pepper

➢ 1/8 teaspoon of ground turmeric

➢ 1/8 teaspoon of ground cinnamon

➢ 1 teaspoon of maple syrup

➢ 1 teaspoon of apple cider vinegar

➢ 2 cups of boiling water

Directions:

1. Pour the boiling water into a small saucepan, add and stir the ginger, then let it rest for 8 to 10 minutes, before covering the pan.

2. Pass the mixture through a strainer and into the liquid, add the cayenne pepper, turmeric, cinnamon and stir properly.

3. Add the maple syrup, vinegar, and lemon slice.

4. Add and stir an infused lemon and serve immediately.

Nutrition: Calories 443 Carbs: 9.7 g Protein: 62.8g Fat: 16.9g

Warm Spiced Lemon Drink

Prep Time:10 minutes

Cook Time:2 hours

Servings: 12

Ingredients:

- ➢ 1 cinnamon stick, about 3 inches long
- ➢ 1/2 teaspoon of whole cloves
- ➢ 2 cups of coconut sugar
- ➢ 4 fluid of ounce pineapple juice
- ➢ 1/2 cup and 2 tablespoons of lemon juice
- ➢ 12 fluid ounce of orange juice
- ➢ 2 1/2 quarts of water

Directions:

1. Pour water into a 6-quarts slow cooker and stir the sugar and lemon juice properly.
2. Wrap the cinnamon, the whole cloves in cheesecloth and tie its corners with string.
3. Immerse this cheesecloth bag in the liquid present in the slow cooker and cover it with the lid.
4. Then plug in the slow cooker and let it cook on high heat setting for 2 hours or until it is heated thoroughly.
5. When done, discard the cheesecloth bag and serve the drink hot or cold.

Nutrition: Calories 523 Carbohydrates: 4.6g Protein: 47.9g Fat: 34.8g

Banana Weight Loss Juice

Prep Time:10 Minutes

Cook Time:0 Minutes

Servings: 1

Ingredients:

- Water (1/3 C.)
- Apple (1, Sliced)
- Orange (1, Sliced)
- Banana (1, Sliced)
- Lemon Juice (1 T.)

Directions:

1. Looking to boost your weight loss? The key is taking in less calories; this recipe can get you there.

2. Simply place everything into your blender, blend on high for twenty seconds, and then pour into your glass.

Nutrition: Calories: 289 Total Carbohydrate: 2 g Cholesterol: 3 mg Total Fat: 17 g Fiber: 2 g Protein: 7 g Sodium: 163 mg

Citrus Detox Juice

Prep Time:10 Minutes

Cook Time:0 Minutes

Servings: 4

Ingredients:

➢ Water (3 C.)

➢ Lemon (1, Sliced)

➢ Grapefruit (1, Sliced)

➢ Orange (1, Sliced)

Directions:

1. While starting your new diet, it is going to be vital to stay hydrated. This detox juice is the perfect solution and offers some extra flavor.

2. Begin by peeling and slicing up your fruit. Once this is done, place in a pitcher of water and infuse the water overnight.

Nutrition: Calories: 269 Total Carbohydrate: 2 g Cholesterol: 3 mg Total Fat: 14 g Fiber: 2 g Protein: 7 g Sodium: 183 mg

Stress Relief Detox Drink

Prep Time:5 Minutes

Cook Time:0 Minutes

Servings: 1

Ingredients:

- ➢ Water (1 Pitcher)
- ➢ Mint
- ➢ Lemon (1, Sliced)
- ➢ Basil
- ➢ Strawberries (1 C., Sliced)
- ➢ Ice

Directions:

1. Life can be a pretty stressful event. Luckily, there is water to help keep you cool, calm, and collected! The lemon works like an energizer, the basil is a natural antidepressant, and mint can help your stomach do its job better. As for the strawberries, those are just for some sweetness!

2. When you are ready, take all of the ingredients and place into a pitcher of water overnight and enjoy the next day.

Nutrition: Calories: 189 Total Carbohydrate: 2 g Cholesterol: 73 mg Total Fat: 17 g Fiber: 0 g Protein: 7 g Sodium: 163 mg

Strawberry Pink Drink

Prep Time:10 Minutes

Cook Time:5 Minutes

Servings: 4

Ingredients:

➢ Water (1 C., Boiling)

➢ Sugar (2 T.)

➢ Acai Tea Bag (1)

➢ Coconut Milk (1 C.)

➢ Frozen Strawberries (1/2 C.)

Directions:

1. If you are looking for a little treat, this is going to be the recipe for you! You will begin by boiling your cup of water and seep the tea bag in for at least five minutes.

2. When the tea is set, add in the sugar and coconut milk. Be sure to stir well to spread the sweetness throughout the tea.

3. Finally, add in your strawberries, and you can enjoy your freshly made pink drink!

Nutrition: Calories: 321 Total Carbohydrate: 2 g Cholesterol: 13 mg Total Fat: 17 g Fiber: 2 g Protein: 9 g Sodium: 312 mg

Almond Butter Brownies

Prep Time:10 minutes

Cook Time:20 minutes

Servings: 4

Ingredients:

- ➢ 1 scoop protein powder
- ➢ 2 tbsp. cocoa powder
- ➢ 1/2 cup almond butter, melted
- ➢ 1 cup bananas, overripe

Directions:

1. Preheat the oven to 350 F/ 176 C.
1. Spray brownie tray with cooking spray.
2. Add all ingredients into the blender and blend until smooth.
3. Pour batter into the prepared dish and bake in preheated oven for 20 minutes.
4. Serve and enjoy.

Nutrition: Calories: 214 Total Carbohydrate: 2 g Cholesterol: 73 mg Total Fat: 7 g Fiber: 2g Protein: 19 g Sodium: 308 g

Quick Chocó Brownie

Prep Time:10 minutes

Cook Time:2 minutes

Servings: 1

Ingredients:

- 1/4 cup almond milk
- 1 tbsp. cocoa powder
- 1 scoop chocolate protein powder
- 1/2 tsp baking powder

Directions:

1. In a microwave-safe mug blend together baking powder, protein powder, and cocoa.
2. Add almond milk in a mug and stir well.
3. Place mug in microwave and microwave for 30 seconds.
4. Serve and enjoy.

Nutrition: Calories: 231 Total Carbohydrate: 2 g Cholesterol: 13 mg Total Fat: 15 g Fiber: 2 g Protein: 8 g Sodium: 298 mg

Coconut Peanut Butter Fudge

Prep Time:1 hour 15 minutes

Cook Time:0 minute

Servings: 20

Ingredients:

- 12 oz. smooth peanut butter
- 3 tbsp. coconut oil
- 4 tbsp. coconut cream
- 15 drops liquid stevia
- Pinch of salt

Directions:

1. Line baking tray with parchment paper.
2. Melt coconut oil in a saucepan over low heat.
3. Add peanut butter, coconut cream, stevia, and salt in a saucepan. Stir well.
4. Pour fudge mixture into the prepared baking tray and place in refrigerator for 1 hour.
5. Cut into pieces and serve.

Nutrition: Calories: 189 Total Carbohydrate: 2 g Cholesterol: 13 mg Total Fat: 7 g Fiber: 2 g Protein: 10 g Sodium: 301 mg

Lemon Mousse

Prep Time:10 minutes

Cook Time:0 minute

Servings: 2

Ingredients:

- ➢ 14 oz. coconut milk
- ➢ 12 drops liquid stevia
- ➢ 1/2 tsp lemon extract
- ➢ 1/4 tsp turmeric

Directions:

1. Place coconut milk can in the refrigerator for overnight. Scoop out thick cream into a mixing bowl.
2. Add remaining ingredients to the bowl and whip using a hand mixer until smooth.
3. Transfer mousse mixture to a zip-lock bag and pipe into small serving glasses. Place in refrigerator.
4. Serve chilled and enjoy.

Nutrition: Calories: 189 Total Carbohydrate: 2 g Cholesterol: 13 mg Total Fat: 7 g Fiber: 2 g Protein: 15 g Sodium: 321 mg

Chocó Chia Pudding

Prep Time:10 minutes

Cook Time:0 minutes

Servings: 6

Ingredients:

- 2 1/2 cups coconut milk
- 2 scoops stevia extract powder
- 6 tbsp. cocoa powder
- 1/2 cup chia seeds
- 1/2 tsp vanilla extract
- 1/8 cup xylitol
- 1/8 tsp salt

Directions:

1. Add all ingredients into the blender and blend until smooth.
2. Pour mixture into the glass container and place in refrigerator.
3. Serve chilled and enjoy.

Nutrition: Calories: 178 Total Carbohydrate: 3 g Cholesterol: 3 mg Total Fat: 17 g Fiber: g Protein: 9 g Sodium: 297 mg

Spiced Buttermilk

Prep Time:5 minutes

Cook Time:0 minute

Servings: 2

Ingredients:

- ➤ 3/4 teaspoon ground cumin
- ➤ 1/4 teaspoon sea salt
- ➤ 1/8 teaspoon ground black pepper
- ➤ 2 mint leaves
- ➤ 1/8 teaspoon lemon juice
- ➤ ¼ cup cilantro leaves
- ➤ 1 cup of chilled water
- ➤ 1 cup vegan yogurt, unsweetened
- ➤ Ice as needed

Directions:

1. Place all the ingredients in the order in a food processor or blender, except for cilantro and ¼ teaspoon cumin, and then pulse for 2 to 3 minutes at high speed until smooth.
2. Pour the milk into glasses, top with cilantro and cumin, and then serve.

Nutrition: Calories: 211 Total Carbohydrate: 7 g Cholesterol: 13 mg Total Fat: 18 g Fiber: 3 g Protein: 17 g Sodium: 289 mg

Soothing Ginger Tea Drink

Prep Time:5 minutes

Cook Time:2 hours 20 minutes

Servings: 8

Ingredients:

➢ 1 tablespoon of minced gingerroot

➢ 2 tablespoons of honey

➢ 15 green tea bags

➢ 32 fluid ounce of white grape juice

➢ 2 quarts of boiling water

Directions:

1. Pour water into a 4-quarts slow cooker, immerse tea bags, cover the cooker and let stand for 10 minutes.
2. After 10 minutes, remove and discard tea bags and stir in remaining ingredients.
3. Return cover to slow cooker, then plug in and let cook at high heat setting for 2 hours or until heated through.
4. When done, strain the liquid and serve hot or cold.

Nutrition: Calories 232 Carbs: 7.9g Protein: 15.9g Fat: 15.1g

Nice Spiced Cherry Cider

Prep Time:1 hour 5 minutes

Cook Time:3 hours

Servings: 16

Ingredients:

➢ 2 cinnamon sticks, each about 3 inches long

➢ 6-ounce of cherry gelatin

➢ 4 quarts of apple cider

Directions:

1. Using a 6-quarts slow cooker, pour the apple cider and add the cinnamon stick.

2. Stir, then cover the slow cooker with its lid. Plug in the cooker and let it cook for 3 hours at the high heat setting or until it is heated thoroughly.

3. Then add and stir the gelatin properly, then continue cooking for another hour.

4. When done, remove the cinnamon sticks and serve the drink hot or cold.

Nutrition: Calories 78 Carbs: 13.2g Protein: 2.8g Fat: 1.5g

Fragrant Spiced Coffee

Prep Time:10 minutes

Cook Time:3 hours

Servings: 8

Ingredients:

- ➢ 4 cinnamon sticks, each about 3 inches long
- ➢ 1 1/2 teaspoons of whole cloves
- ➢ 1/3 cup of honey
- ➢ 2-ounce of chocolate syrup
- ➢ 1/2 teaspoon of anise extract
- ➢ 8 cups of brewed coffee

Directions:

1. Pour the coffee in a 4-quarts slow cooker and pour in the remaining ingredients except for cinnamon and stir properly.
2. Wrap the whole cloves in cheesecloth and tie its corners with strings.
3. Immerse this cheesecloth bag in the liquid present in the slow cooker and cover it with the lid.
4. Then plug in the slow cooker and let it cook on the low heat setting for 3 hours or until heated thoroughly.
5. When done, discard the cheesecloth bag and serve.

Nutrition: Calories 136 Fat 12.6 g Carbohydrates 4.1 g Sugar 0.5 g Protein 10.3 g Cholesterol 88 mg

Inspirational Orange Smoothie

Prep Time:5 minutes

Cook Time:5 minutes

Servings: 1

Ingredients:

➢ 4 mandarin oranges, peeled

➢ 1 banana, sliced and frozen

➢ ½ cup non-fat Greek yoghurt

➢ ¼ cup coconut water

➢ 1 tsp vanilla extract

➢ 5 ice cubes

Directions:

1. Using a mixer, whisk all the ingredients.

2. Enjoy your drink!

Nutrition: Calories 256 Fat 13.3 g Carbohydrates 0 g Sugar 0 g Protein 34.5 g Cholesterol 78 mg

High Protein Blueberry Banana Smoothie

Prep Time:5 minutes

Cook Time:5 minutes

Servings: 2

Ingredients:

- ➢ 1 cup blueberries, frozen
- ➢ 2 ripe bananas
- ➢ 1 cup water
- ➢ 1 tsp vanilla extract
- ➢ 2 Tbsp. chia seeds
- ➢ ½ cup cottage cheese
- ➢ 1 tsp lemon zest

Directions:

1. Put all the smoothie ingredients into the blender and whisk until smooth.
2. Enjoy your wonderful smoothie!

Nutrition: Calories 358 Fat 19.8 g Carbohydrates 1.3 g Sugar 0.4 g Protein 41.9 g Cholesterol 131 mg

Ginger Smoothie with Citrus and Mint

Prep Time:5 minutes

Cook Time:3 minutes

Servings: 3

Ingredients:

➤ 1 head Romaine lettuce, chopped into 4 chunks

➤ 2 Tbsp. hemp seeds

➤ 5 mandarin oranges, peeled

➤ 1 banana, frozen

➤ 1 carrot

➤ 2-3 mint leaves

➤ ½ piece ginger root, peeled

➤ 1 cup water

➤ ¼ lemon, peeled

➤ ½ cup ice

Directions:

1. Put all the smoothie ingredients in a blender and blend until smooth.

2. Enjoy!

Nutrition: Calories 101 Fat 4 g Carbohydrates 14 g Sugar 1 g Protein 2 g Cholesterol 3 mg

Strawberry Beet Smoothie

Prep Time: 5 minutes

Cook Time: 50 minutes

Servings: 2

Ingredients:

➢ 1 red beet, trimmed, peeled and chopped into cubes

➢ 1 cup strawberries, quartered

➢ 1 ripe banana

➢ ½ cup strawberry yoghurt

➢ 1 Tbsp. honey

➢ 1 Tbsp. water

➢ Milk, to taste

Directions:

1. Sprinkle the beet cubes with water, place on aluminum foil and put in the oven (preheated to 204°C). Bake for 40 minutes.

2. Let the baked beet cool.

3. Combine all the smoothie ingredients.

4. Enjoy your fantastic drink.

Nutrition: Calories 184 Fat 9.2 g Carbohydrates 1 g Sugar 0.4 g Protein 24.9 g Cholesterol 132 mg

Peanut Butter Shake

Prep Time:5 minutes

Cook Time:5 minutes

Servings: 2

Ingredients:

- ➢ 1 cup plant-based milk
- ➢ 1 handful kale
- ➢ 2 bananas, frozen
- ➢ 2 Tbsp. peanut butter
- ➢ ½ tsp ground cinnamon
- ➢ ¼ tsp vanilla powder

Directions:

1. Use a blender to combine all the ingredients for your shake.

2. Enjoy it!

Nutrition: Calories 184 Fat 9.2 g Carbohydrates 1 g Sugar 0.4 g Protein 24.9 g Cholesterol 132 mg

Lightning Source UK Ltd.
Milton Keynes UK
UKHW021833040621
384966UK00002B/471

9 781802 857764